*Life-giving Intervention
Along Life's Path Occurs*

When Jesus
Shows Up

*A Nurse's Testimony of God's
Healing on the Job*

SUSAN SCHUNEMANN NORRIS

◆ FriesenPress

Suite 300 - 990 Fort St
Victoria, BC, V8V 3K2
Canada

www.friesenpress.com

ISBN
978-1-03-911210-0 (Hardcover)
978-1-03-911209-4 (Paperback)
978-1-03-911211-7 (eBook)

1. *Body, Mind & Spirit, Healing, Prayer & Spiritual*

Distributed to the trade by The Ingram Book Company

TABLE OF CONTENTS

Dedication

I dedicate this book to my husband, Jake, who has encouraged me along the way, and my entire family and all their children.

God Bless families everywhere that are searching for more love, harmony and healing. May the door open for Jesus to show up increasingly in all our lives until the trumpet sounds and we shall see him face to face.

INTRODUCTION

My journey in nursing all started with a prayer and a promise.

I was taught early on in my training that nursing is a vocation. It is a calling. That realization did not become evident to me until much later, when I had to console the inconsolable, encourage those paralyzed with fear and forgive the angry souls whose words could knock me to the ground.

It was New Years Eve 1988 at a celebration in the home where I attended a bible fellowship every week. As during every New Years Eve, I wanted to think about what direction I could possibly go in the upcoming year. This year was special—I was truly at a crossroads. I was living alone at the time and working where there was no career advancement, trying to make it by as best I could. I was living in a different part of the country from the rest of my family, and the questions were, should I move, change jobs, where should I go and what should I do in order to move forward?

1

I stepped away from my friends in the kitchen into a small den and sat on the sofa. There it was quiet and I was alone in the room. I just prayed a heartfelt prayer to God on this New Years Eve—thanking Him for opening doors of opportunity, and more importantly, having the courage to walk through them.

A few months went by and a friend of mine began telling me about a job opening in registration at the local hospital where she was working, and it sounded like a good place to start my new journey. Maybe eventually it could be a springboard into other areas. After just a few months of working at the registration desk, I had observed patients of all ages, with a variety of physical problems, many of which were life threatening.

I was so moved by their plights, vulnerabilities, and suffering, that a desire to do more for them besides just filling out their forms, continued to grow.

That summer of 1989, a wide door of opportunity presented itself. The hospital was experiencing a nursing shortage and the administrators wanted to offer twelve nursing scholarships to qualifying applicants. There was a buzz around the department as to who would apply and who would get in.

I had to ask myself, "Do I want to do this?" Going back to school was a huge commitment. Yet, if I made up my mind to move forward with this, I knew in my heart there would be no turning back. There, in front of me stood the open door that I had prayed for months before, and then I remembered that I also prayed for the courage to go through it, as well.

The scholarship came like a gift. Everything would be paid for, and all I had to do was work two 8 hour shifts at the hospital as a nursing assistant and get a "C" average in all the classes. In turn, I would receive a weekly paycheck for 40 hours of work! So, let's see, I would have time to study in the evenings, money for all my expenses, tuition paid for, and all my books paid for. What a Godsend!

So, that is how the journey started. I understand that God's timing is perfect, and I later learned that the year those scholarships were handed out, was the only time in the hospital's history that they were ever given.

CHAPTER 1

Miracles, Mothers and Newborns

Hebrews 4:16 NIV

"Let us then approach God's throne of grace with confidence so that we may receive mercy and find grace to help us in our time of need."

After I graduated the nursing program and had license in hand, my first assignment was to work in the Women's Care Center.

Sounded good to me, shouldn't be too overwhelming for a very green nurse, such as myself. I was indebted to work a few years at the hospital that paid my tuition, and this is where I landed.

It was a busy morning that day in the Women's Care Center, and I usually had six or seven patients during a 12-hour shift.

There were quite a variety of surgeries and conditions on the floor, ranging from breast biopsies to cervical radiation implants, ovarian cancer complications requiring radical surgical intervention and, of course, the mothers recovering from cesarian section. Also, there were mothers who were placed separately from the rest of the mother/baby population, after having miscarriage, stillborn, or those whose infants were needing care in the neonatal intensive care unit. This was the case of the patient I was about to receive from labor hall.

She was, of course, a young woman, still groggy from the medications given during the emergency cesarean section that she just underwent. I was told from the reporting nurse that her labor was difficult, the baby was in severe distress and during labor, inhaled a large amount of fluid mixed with its own stool. As the baby was lifted from the mother during the c-section, the air transport personnel were standing by waiting to whisk it away to the nearest NICU. For the infant to need air transport to a hospital in the same city, it had to be critical.

To make the situation so much more painful for the mother—she was never given the opportunity to see the baby, hold the baby or even hear his cry.

As she lay there quietly, semi-conscious from sedation, her assessment was normal. I checked all the necessary criteria that ensured she was recovering without complications.

And so ended her day of surgery, and hopefully, she could quickly be reunited with her precious newborn within a couple of days.

Upon returning the next morning to the Women's Care Center, there were assigned to me a group of patients a little further down the hall, and I was hoping that I still had Mrs. Wellington, the new mom, but she was in a different group with a different nurse.

After receiving report on my patients, I went to my co-worker, Darla, who was now in charge of Mrs. Wellington's care, and asked how she fared through the night. This was a great, caring team of professionals at the hospital back then, and we all continued to have a genuine interest in the well-being of our patients, even after they were discharged and sent home!

Many were young cancer patients that we were all rooting for and bonded with during their hospital stay.

To my dismay, Mrs. Wellington developed a blood clot in her right calf-and now had to remain bedridden for eleven more days on intravenous blood thinners. How was she going to feel about this? She hadn't even seen her baby yet! I just had to figure out a time to slip into her room and check on her-give her a kind word, anything!

About mid-morning I quietly walked into her room—she was awake and was dabbing her eyes with a tissue. Her red rimmed, swollen eyes met mine as I asked how she was. Pointing to her right leg, I saw the edema in her lower calf and the circular pink area on her skin above the location of the DVT or deep vein thrombosis.

She was scared and panicky at the prospect at being "stuck here" —away from her newborn. I could only imagine. I just had to do something…I turned my head to see past the open door, and there was her internist standing at the nurse's station, leaning on the counter, busily writing in a chart.

I wanted to check with him, see what he had to say about her dilemma. When asked about the blood clot, he answered, without looking up from her chart, "Oh, yes," he replied quickly, "the way things are going for her, I wouldn't be surprised if it (blood clot) broke off, like everything else that has gone wrong." His words jolted me. If that were to happen, her life could end very quickly and there would be nothing any of us could do.

Ok, I thought to myself, I have confirmation that she has an immediate need and I am going to have to do something.

A rush of excitement and nervousness went through me. This was gearing up to be one of those moments when heaven and earth would collide.

I walked back in. If ever I saw a woman at the end of her rope, this was it. The head of her bed was about halfway up, her face in her hands, sobbing almost uncontrollably. "I have to see my baby"

She certainly did—but here she was with a life-threatening clot that required her to be here in the bed for eleven more days!

Her sobs were a primordial, heartfelt cry from the deepest chamber in a woman's heart—a cry for her baby in trouble, yet all the while having arms that could not reach it, arms that could not hold it, and arms that could not comfort it.

I could feel her heart breaking, and then, an inner strength stirred in me. There was only one thing at that pivotal moment in time that I could do. It did not involve any sedatives, counseling or comfort measures. Only one thing to do, which was to take her by the hand, and lead her into the throne room of God's grace.

"Mrs. Wellington," taking her hands in mine, "you need a miracle."

"Do you believe God can heal?"

"Yes, yes! I do! "she answered without hesitation. Still holding her hands in mine, I said with authority, "Well then, we're going to pray."

Ok, I thought, here it goes! "Father, in the name of Jesus Christ, I claim healing in Mrs. Wellington's body-that the clot in her leg be dissolved right now—in the powerful name of Jesus Christ."

She took a deep breath, wiped her eyes, was visibly calm. As if right on cue, two technicians strode into her room with a stretcher, helping her slide onto it. "What are we doing now?" I inquired.

"Just taking her to ultrasound to measure the DVT"….and off she went down the hall to the elevator.

So, I went about my business, and then, no more than thirty minutes later—I see a stretcher being wheeled out of the elevator with a technician at each end starting to bring it back down the hall.

Sitting straight up in the middle of the stretcher— a young woman with raised arms outstretched in victory—speaking with an overflowing joy echoing down the hall…"Susan, it's gone!"

It was amazing how quickly her discharge papers were drawn up-her nurse had her IV removed, and a wheelchair was brought in. Just like the way her baby was whisked away from her, she was being whisked right back to him. Within an hour from the time we prayed together, she was at her baby's side.

They were both back at home soon after.

What I will never forget is the joy radiating from that woman, as she sat up in the stretcher, coming back down the hall, arms outstretched in victory.

CHAPTER 1

The Treasure of a Sound Mind

2 Timothy 1:7 KJB

"For God hath not given us a spirit of fear, but of power, and love, and of a sound mind."

When I took the staff nurse position on an acute care psychiatric floor, I began to observe an entirely different kind of suffering than what I was used to seeing. Most of these patients didn't have any broken bones or surgical pain, but their wounds were buried beneath the surface of their skin, and the havoc these conditions wreaked in their lives was far more debilitating.

There were alcoholics bent on self-destruction, bipolar patients with mood swings so severe that one took a shotgun to his own beloved horse and shot it in a fit of rage. There were spending sprees that wives would get caught up in, leaving insurmountable debts, causing life-long burdens in their wake. These were just a few of the afflictions that patients were admitted with.

One day, I observed a man being admitted with psychosis. He was standing at the nurses' station, leaning on his elbows with his face in his hands, sobbing, exhausted, tormented. He had no control over the voices in his head. He was terrified that they were directing him to the fast-food restaurant down the street and ordering him to shoot the customers inside. His voice was shaky and weak. What if he couldn't stop himself, he agonized.

At that moment, I realized that having a sound mind was something that up until that moment, I had taken for granted. Oh, what a thing to be treasured and thankful for! Quiet, peaceful thoughts, the ability to focus on what we choose and to dwell on those things that build us up. My life was changed forever that day, I would never see the verse of scripture in 2 Timothy 1:7 in the same way. Now I had an appreciation for just how unsound a mind can get. I will see the words, "For God hath not given us the spirit of fear, but of power, and of love, and of a sound mind" in capital letters!

Most of the battles we engage in take place in the mind. This is where we can triumph in life, where we can defeat the evil trying to germinate in the form of thoughts. Thoughts of failure can be replaced with thoughts of success, and fears replaced with love. God has not given us the spirit of fear, the bible says, but of power…yes, power.

Her room was across from the nurses' station, and she was brought in the night before by her family. Depression, left untreated, can render a person unable to function. At all. I was busy getting organized for the morning and the social worker had already begun the morning group discussion in the main activity room. All the patients were in attendance, except for the most recent admission, my new patient, I will call Brenda. I looked up from my desk through the plexiglass partition, across the hall and into Brenda's room. There she lay—on the floor, facing up toward the ceiling, listless, devoid of any motivation or energy. I had read in school where infants that are left uncared for, with physical touch withheld, can become so depressed that they just lie motionless, so completely, that flies can land on their unblinking eyes.

Brenda needed to be liberated, to be made free. This depression was exterminating the life from her.

I walked into the room and looked down toward her expressionless face and motionless body. I knelt down on the floor beside her. She did not acknowledge my presence in any way. I reached out and touched her shoulder speaking very softly. I felt compassion welling up inside me for this tortured soul. I was inspired to speak of the love of Jesus, and the love that he had for her. Quietly, I kept giving her words of hope and reassurance. At this point, her eyes turned towards me, and were now becoming focused. I held her hand, and in just as soft a voice, commanded the depression to leave her, then took her by the hand, and without any further words, she got up off the floor and into the shower. After she showered, she proceeded to get ready for the day; quietly and slowly, but cooperatively.

Here was a woman who had been in a trance-like state for two weeks. She ate lunch, and much to my joy, walked into the afternoon group therapy session. Afterwards, I asked the therapist how Brenda was getting along. She reported to me that Brenda participated in the discussion and "did OK." She seemed a little puzzled at my great joy over what seemed to her as normal behavior during a group session. But then again, she did not witness the change in Brenda—the miraculous change from a catatonic state to an alert, cooperative, functioning individual in just a moment of time. Why?

Because there is power in the love of Jesus.

CHAPTER 3

God Is Light—A Young Mother's Hope

John 5:6 KJV

"When Jesus saw him lie, and knew that he had been now a long time in that case, he saith unto him,

Wilt thou be made whole?"

Sitting alone in her hospital room, Alice was far from her home in southeastern Kentucky. Like many other women in the surrounding counties who were suffering from gynecological cancers, she sought treatment on the women's floor where I worked as a registered nurse.

Alice's story was one of great adversity, and in the face of it all, her humility and quiet, serene disposition remained on an even keel.

Tonight, she was going to have her husband drive up with their twin boys so they could spend some much- needed time with mom. The visit would be a significant moment in the life of Alice because of the potentially life-altering surgery she had schedule for the following morning. Her role as caregiver to her boys was threatened to be changed forever.

A couple of years before, she had radiation treatments to her pelvic area to halt the spread of cervical cancer.

In Alice's case, a complication occurred when those treatments damaged the surrounding arteries, severely compromising the circulation to both legs.

Doctors and technicians were in and out of her room all day, discussing the surgery, prepping her for what needed to be done, but told her that the outcome was not looking good, considering the amount of damage done in both femoral arteries.

The surgeons were going to attempt to repair the severely damaged arteries, and if unsuccessful, both legs would have to be amputated at the hip.

So, that was the plan, and that was the horrific scenario that was laid out before her.

Shortly after this heavy burden was delivered, her little twin boys, seven years old, showed up with their dad.

They were so eager and happy to see her, all dressed up in their little cub scout uniforms. Their innocence, their vulnerability, stole the heart of all the nurses.

One could not imagine by observing Alice that there was a weight on Alice's shoulders as she interacted with her children, smiling and attentive to their excited chatter of all the news from home.

After they hugged and kissed good-bye, her husband bravely walked with the boys to the elevator, and as the doors closed behind them, they disappeared from view.

Down on the first floor, an arched opening led into the main lobby where patients and visitors passed as they entered and exited the hospital. An inscription above the arch read, "Wilt thou be made whole?"

How perfect was that, I thought, to quote Jesus and pose the question to all those in need of wholeness.

Jesus was asking the infirm man in John 5:6 if he had the will to be healed.

I turned to Alice's room to see if she needed anything and how she was faring. Our conversation was relaxed and easy. She talked about her church, her relationship with God, but unfortunately was not aware of the scriptures regarding healing in His children. She was not sure that she could count on God to see her through, and in her mind, doubt, worry and fear were creeping in.

I suggested that at times when we needed something short and easy to remember, like a mantra, we can hinge our thoughts upon it to get us through a rough patch.

She totally agreed. Knowing that she was a God rev-erencing woman, and that God's word carries spirit and life with it, I offered her a simple, yet power-packed scripture from 1 John 1:5.

"God is light and in Him in no darkness at all."

She readily received that, and we repeated it together several times, so I was sure that she "had it down."

The worry on her face was transformed into a calm, trusting demeanor as she focused on this simple truth of 1 John 1:5 that said so much in so few words.

The next morning as I came on duty, she was already in surgery. Like Alice, I was just going to focus on God being light and that He wills only good things for our lives.

Some hours later, the surgeons on her case were strolling down the hall in their surgical scrubs, high fiving each other! I took this as good news…Not long after that, here comes Alice on a gurney, with such serenity, such peace.

After she was settled in her room, she eagerly reported to me her experience.

As the surgical technicians rolled her to surgery, her only view as she lay on her back, were the ceiling tiles, rolling by one by one, keeping rhythm with the mantra she was repeating, "God is light and in Him is no dark-ness at all."

Upon awakening, the first thing she did was reach with her hands and feel for her legs. Her heart was then filled with praise for the God of the impossible, the one in whom she placed her trust, as she could feel both her legs, still there, intact.

And so, she was joyfully able to walk out of the hospital, with a deeper understanding and trust in a loving God, and to experience His healing touch, through His son, Jesus.

And the question Jesus posed in John 5:6, "Wilt thou be made whole?" will always remain, to all of us seeking the Healer's touch, a critical issue of introspection that must be answered with all honesty.

The sick man that Jesus was addressing was in a weakened condition for a long time. Had he lost the desire to get better? Where was his expectation?

Did he have the will, after all this time, to be healed?

For Alice, just like the man in the gospel of John, the answer was a resounding "YES.

CHAPTER 4

He Took Even That
to the Cross

Psalm 34:18 NIV

"The Lord is close to the brokenhearted and saves those who are crushed in spirit."

"Abdominal Pain" was the reason given on her emergency room report as to why she was here, which was supposed to be just an overnight stay.

I caught a glimpse of her being rolled in a wheelchair down the hallway to her room. A young woman at her side was carrying the overnight bag, and the patient, an older woman, had her eyes cast downward, hunching forward in the wheelchair. She did seem in distress, almost as if she were shrouded by a dark cloud.

OK, I thought, better get on this and get her settled and checked in. I brought the usual items with me for admission: hospital gown, socks, blanket, toiletries, etc.

The patient, whom I will call Betty, was sitting in a chair near the bed, and across from her sat her daughter, Pam.

Betty, who was in her sixties, with short, dark hair and a kind face that was now tear stained and eyes that reflected loads of pain.

When I asked her about that, she replied that the pain had subsided and that a colonoscopy was scheduled later that week. She continued dabbing her eyes and going through one tissue after another. Pam drew near to her, placing an arm around her shoulders and then looked at me.

"My mom is very upset; her husband of forty-two years came home from work today with the news that he is leaving her. There's another woman." And just like that, he was gone.

Pam seemed in shock and Betty was breaking in pieces before me. She stood up and started walking back and forth, sobbing and choking with grief. Raw betrayal, the inhumanity of it, I thought. They were both willing to talk, it was like a release for them. No, they did not have a forewarning—this was just dropped on both right out of the blue. Forty-two years married that is a long time. While Betty is looking forward to retirement, spending time with her husband and family, she very suddenly found herself rejected by him, cast mercilessly aside, lost and bewildered.

Surely, just telling her, "I'm sorry, hope it all works out," seemed so trite and empty. If I could just point her in the direction of the one who can really heal the brokenhearted—that would be the best.

So, I asked them if they had heard of Jesus, if they believed in God. Enthusiastically, they answered yes, they had faith and believed in God.

Standing here were His people, stabbed in the heart in one of the most painful ways—betrayal. How critical it was that they were reminded of God's love and desire to see them through this ordeal with His strength.

I remember how their eyes were so glued on me with rapt attention as I spoke those healing words from Psalm 147:3. "He heals the brokenhearted and binds up their wounds"

And now, the important truth to accept fully, is how Jesus took every sin against us, including her betrayal, and nailed it to that cross on that day. He truly is the heavy lifter of all our sorrows. (Isaiah 53:4a "Surely he hath borne our griefs, and carried our sorrows")

It was as if the heaviness was being lifted, they were no longer slumped in their chairs, but sitting up straight. New determination to beat this thing started to come alive in their conversation. They talked about going back to be with their church family and reminding each other of the need for the presence of God in their lives. Their conversation was sounding more like excited chatter-an awakening. It showed in the softening of their facial expressions and the de-escalation of their fury. At that moment I knew that they would walk through this and they would not fall into the pit of despair. How we need to remind each other of these great truths, and they are truly a shield and buckler to all those who live by them.

So, Betty and Pam were now in position to walk through this chapter of their lives, not just by being strong by themselves, but as the word directs....

"Be strong in the LORD and in the power of HIS might."

Their faces reflected determination to rise, and with their Lord's help, move forward.

Once they had this new resolve, they were ready to go back home. Betty had no symptoms at this point, so she was able to be discharged soon after.

I saw the nursing assistant rolling her wheelchair by the desk, only this time, she had a smile, and a wave goodbye. In that genuine smile, there was a new outlook on life. With her lord's help, she would rise and move forward.

It never ceases to amaze me how transforming the word of God is. One can move from lost to found, hopeless to hopeful, and despairing to encouraged, in just the time it takes to hear the promise of God and embrace it.

Hebrews 4:12 KJV

"For the word of God is quick and powerful, and sharper than any two-edged sword, piercing even to the dividing asunder of soul and spirit, and of the joints and marrow, and is a discerner of the thoughts and intents of the heart."

CHAPTER 5

Never Alone

Proverbs 18:24 NIV

"One who has unreliable friends soon comes to ruin, but there is a friend who sticks closer than a brother."

It was Christmas time, and I was working in a home for the elderly, the infirm, veterans from World War 11 era, often referred to as the greatest generation, and I could see why. Some of the residents had survived the landing at Normandy Beach, others had survived the front lines in Nazi Germany, and a few had flown missions all over western Europe. They had survived unthinkable obstacles against all odds. Many had spent four years in combat and were now in their sunset years. These were the men I was privileged to care for.

One resident comes to mind. He was not even a shadow of his former self. His body was twisted and bent. He was unable to speak at all.

His wife came in every day faithfully, and she always seemed to know what he needed and when he needed it.

She could look into his bright blue eyes and give him a drink of water or reposition him in his geriatric chair. One day, she placed a photograph of the two of them standing together dressed elegantly taken many years before, and I was shocked. How could this be the same man, I thought? He stood so tall, was so handsome. I learned he was the former CEO of a very large greeting card company, but as time went by he became increasingly infirm, bringing him to the condition he was in at the time I met him.

Though married for over fifty years, Mrs. Courtney, as I will call her, couldn't stay in the same residence with her beloved, going home every night, alone.

She was a petite woman, yet always found the physical strength to lift and turn him, change and feed him, day after day. How I admired her courage and devotion.

Now, it was Christmas Eve, and I was anticipating a nice evening at home with my husband, where we would share a home cooked meal and then exchange gifts.

I put on my winter coat, grabbed my purse, and headed down the corridor towards the parking lot. I was newly married at the time, and having someone special to share the holidays with, was something I was especially thankful for.

Before this time in my life, there were several years that I celebrated the holidays without a companion, yet I honestly never really felt alone….

Rounding the corner of the building, I saw a familiar form, wrapped in a warm coat, slowly making her way to the car. It was Mrs. Courtney. I slowed to her pace and began engaging her in conversation.

"No," she admitted to me, "I don't enjoy the holidays like I used to. My children are grown and moved away, and I am alone at the house. Most holidays I stay home so I can come back and take care of Ted, but the nights I am alone." I could just feel the sadness in her heart. I understood that the holidays could leave many people with the impression that they are missing out if their calendars are not filled with dinner invitations with friends and family surrounding them.

Awhile back, I learned about a truly different approach to celebrating, a way of making Christmas and New Year's special without the fanfare. It actually gave a sense of well-being and peace, and I found that these quiet nights were nothing to be afraid of. I found it enjoyable, so I went ahead and shared my experience, and she looked at me as a woman who was ready to change her outlook and experience some joy for a change.

"What I like to do," I explained, "is find a quiet time somewhere between Christmas and New Year's, turn the lights down, except for the Christmas lights and just light some candles, maybe enjoy a glass of wine or hot chocolate, and think of all the things that I am thankful for. I like to write in a journal the highlights of the past year and then write down what I would like to see happen in the coming year. As I think about these things, I have a heart-to-heart talk with the one who cares the most, my heavenly Father. Just God and I, peace and quiet, candlelight and heartfelt prayer time, a time of refreshing. I find that it has a great impact on my attitude if I just allow God to love me and I can just bask in His presence."

I looked at Mrs. Courtney's smiling face as if it were just the thing she wanted to try.

A week or so later, when I saw her visiting her husband, she walked up to me, eager to report what a difference there was in her holiday experience this time. She told me that she lit some candles, and closed out the rest of the world, while she and the One matters most had a long overdue heartfelt time together. It was a peaceful and healing time.

What a joy it is to realize that we are never alone.

CHAPTER 6

Encircled with Prayer: Courage in the Face of Cancer

James 5:15 Berean Study Bible

"And the prayer offered in faith will restore the one who is sick. The Lord will raise him up. If he has sinned, he will be forgiven."

Despite the unfavorable outcomes of many with an ovarian cancer diagnosis, the patient I met that morning was calm and composed. She was having surgery later that morning to remove an ovarian tumor and smiled serenely as I walked into her room and introduced myself. I noticed her pale blonde hair and very fair skin tone. She was of Swedish descent, I learned, and was happily awaiting the arrival of her five children, which I assumed had her Nordic features as well. They were traveling from all over the country to see her to surgery and wish her well.

She was going to need it, I thought to myself. We saw lots of cases of ovarian cancer on this surgical oncology unit, and they always had an intense regimen of chemotherapy and over time multiple surgeries. I had been praying to see someone spared of this outcome. Someone who would dare to reach for the impossible, believing that God actually specializes in impossible. I was still waiting.

Today was Mrs. Clemson's big day. She will be going to surgery, where a lot of questions would be answered. I do not recall her speaking much at all, she simply cooperated calmly, no signs of anxiety. The introspective blonde lady waiting for her children to arrive.

When I returned to her room an hour later, she was surrounded by her three sons and two daughters, all so dignified and well dressed. The tone was reverent, hushed-and there was a peace, that made the room inviting. It was the absence of fear that made the whole dynamic different from so many others.

As I looked around the room, I could not help but notice that all five of these children of a very light complected mother were as dark skinned as mahogany, and it surprised me just a little.

Then I saw a picture of her late husband at her bedside, in uniform, tall and handsome like his children, and dark skinned. They had met while he was in the service, and I was sad for her that she was a widow, but the devotion of her children to all be there for her and rally around her was heartwarming.

One of her sons was in his navy uniform-a naval chaplain and was holding the bible in his hands. He stood tall and had a presence that commanded great respect.

I turned toward the door, and the surgical technicians in scrubs walked in pushing a stretcher. One was a petite oriental lady with her hair tucked in a surgical cap, and the other was an older woman also in scrubs. I helped Mrs. Clemson slide over to the stretcher as she moved easily, her family stood attentively by her side. Then someone in the family asked for prayer, and everyone in the room immediately formed a circle around the patient and held hands. It just all happened automatically, silently, as everyone smoothly fell into place. We were all strangers, yet so united in being a part of this special moment. I was wondering who would do the praying, and of course, the naval chaplain began without hesitation. As he invoked the blessings of God, through His son, Jesus Christ upon his mother, I was so touched that seeing all the different nationalities present in the room, from all different backgrounds, could come together in unity of purpose. Everyone's head was bowed in prayer, together in one accord at this time and place.

As soon as the prayer ended, final hugs and encouraging smiles exchanged, everyone dispersed as quickly as they came together, to carry on with their roles in the surgical care of Mrs. Clemson. Her children disappeared to the surgical waiting room, and I tended to my other patients.

During the rest of the afternoon, I kept wondering about how Mrs. Clemson was doing. It was as if I just could not wait to hear how everything went.

When the recovery room nurse called to give me the report, she just said they removed the tumor along with the ovary, but there was a sac around it, like a wall, preventing the cancer from spreading anywhere. Just a completely encapsulating sac, which was removed so easily, no further treatment necessary.

As we encircled her with prayer, the cancer was encircled with a protective wall, and her life was spared from all the medical treatments that would normally be the next step in fighting the cancer battle.

She had a healthy dose of courage, fearlessness, love and faith, and in the end, God was able to deliver her from the snare of this disease, and all those who knew her had great cause for rejoicing.

And His peace ruled.

CHAPTER 7

A Change of Heart

Proverbs 4:23 NIV

"Above all else, guard your heart, for everything you do flows from it."

It was an especially trying time for me in those days, after taking a position at the veterans' home. The facility was located about twenty-five miles away, down winding country roads, which required an extra early start every morning. The facility itself was state of the art, and had a total three hundred bed capacity, having five wings with sixty beds in each wing.

I was the charge nurse in one of those wings, which involved the supervision of the nurses and assistants in that area. Although, the facility was relatively new and well designed, the organization inside was chaotic at best. The supplies were in disarray, the patient rooms were cluttered, with clothing piled everywhere, opened snacks crammed into drawers, and various personal

items that were occupying every inch of free space. The equipment room was cluttered with dirty wheel-chairs, walkers, and various devices. One look told me I was facing a major overhaul of the entire wing in order to restore some semblance of cleanliness and organization.

There was never enough staff—as soon as someone was hired, someone else would take another position, and we were understaffed again. Then, if a nurse called in sick for the oncoming shift, I would have to stay over and work another eight hours if no one else could cover.

Needless to say, I got pretty good at motivating people to work extra. Thankfully, most of them needed the money.

On top of the less-than-ideal working conditions, there were physical and verbal fights taking place amongst the staff! On weekends when I was the head nurse, I would get calls overhead to various departments to step in and intervene when a fight broke out, usually in the kitchen or laundry room. Here, in this neck of the woods, this is how some attempted to solve their differences.

There was also a struggle with my energy waning—especially at the end of the day when I had to drive home. As much as I tried to fight this, I would still start to doze off at a long red light. The windows were rolled down, radio turned up, but still, no match for those long red lights.

About this time, one of the nurse's aides, Anita, approached me with a request. Now Anita had a very colorful personality. She was boisterous, jolly, wore pink-tinged granny glasses, had gold front teeth, and multi-colored dreadlocks. Though she was a little rough around the edges, she was likeable and had a way of making me laugh along with her.

Her request was, could I pick her up on the way to work every morning and drop her off at home every evening after work. She was without wheels and would so appreciate it. Well, I thought, if I do not do this and she cannot get to work, I will be yet another worker short, so no problem, I would do it.

The thing about Anita was that she loved to talk while I drove. She described her life…her childhood in Chicago, her love of cooking, (some of my favorite recipes are from good 'ol Anita), her kids and the trouble they were frequently in. She had no husband, and she and her 2 teenaged sons lived with her daughter and 3 grandchildren in a small townhouse in the south end of town. Sometimes she talked about her two brothers that she hadn't seen in a long while and that she missed them. Where were they? In prison— each serving a life sentence for "murder one."

One thing about Anita, I never had another problem with falling asleep at the wheel as long as she was in the car.

She was a lifesaver. And I learned that everyone has amazing stories and that we never really know the struggles someone may be having under the surface.

It is so important to guard against passing judgement based on the outer appearance.

During this time, I discovered the cause of all the symptoms that I had been enduring for years—the abdominal tenderness, weakness, frequent running to the bathroom. After my doctor ordered a colonoscopy, and the results were in, my doctor called me at home.

I was told that the entire length of my colon was ulcerated due to ulcerative colitis, an autoimmune disease that is progressive. I would need a colostomy in a few years down the road.

Surely it would not ever come to that, I thought. In the meantime, the anti-inflammatory drugs really made a difference, and I was overjoyed at the relief I was given.

However, as the disease was progressive, the oral medication started to become ineffective.

I remembered being told at one time, that if ever one finds themselves in a corner, one can always reach up.

I was at a place where I could sink or swim, in a corner where all I could do was reach up, a crossroads in my faith journey.

I could choose to rely on what medicine could do for me, which was an option, but not the kind of option that appealed to me. With that said, I was still thankful that there was that option should it come down to that.

Or, I could choose to reach up to the God of the impossible, the God who presides over the physical realm, the God who is all light and all love.

Before I reached to Him, I knew that any doubt I may be harboring in my heart regarding victory over this disease-needed to be washed out. How would I accomplish this cleansing? I thought of Psalm 119:9, "Wherewithal shall a young man cleanse his way? By taking heed according to thy word." The word cleanses- it cleanses our minds, our hearts, and ultimately, our lives.

I knew enough about the bible to know that the heart is where our core beliefs, our strongest emotions, our deepest desires and passions lie. If we are going to have a change of heart, we must change the way we believe. It can be done.

The change starts with the thoughts we are feeding our mind. What are we watching, listening to, reading about, and dwelling on? Eventually, what we hold onto in our minds, works its way down into our heart, and becomes part of who we are.

Negative thinking, when allowed to incubate in our minds, turns doubts and worries into actual fears. On the other hand, the opposite is true. When the good news of the teachings of Jesus Christ, and the promises of God are made known to us, then allowed to incubate in our minds and work their way into our hearts, then are we truly made free.

With that in mind, I began to study the last week of Jesus's life, including the crucifixion. There were many things he endured—rejection, betrayal, whippings, beatings, tortures, severe mental pressure—yet innocent of any crimes or wrongdoings. Moreover, he had innocent blood.

Many of his followers at the time did not fully realize that prophecies regarding the coming Messiah, written thousands of years before, were being fulfilled before their eyes. Isaiah 53:5, written seven hundred years earlier, reads, "But he was wounded for our transgressions, he was bruised for our iniquities, the chastisement of our peace was upon him, and with his stripes, we are healed."

He walked in perfect harmony with his father, God, never giving in to temptation. He was all love and loved all. By doing this, he accomplished for us what we could not do for ourselves, and that is, to be reconciled back to God.

It all became so clear to me, by his stripes I am healed.

Will I receive that? Healing is never forced on us. It is written, "Yet, you don't have what you want because you don't ask God for it." James 4:2

"But when you ask him, be sure your faith is in God alone. Do not waiver, for a person with divided loyalty is as unsettled as a wave of the sea, that is blown and tossed by the wind." James 1:6

I stood by the sliding glass doors in the dining room. I had made up my mind. If there was anyone on the planet that did not want Jesus to have gone through all those temptations, tortures and sacrifice of his life that he willingly gave at his crucifixion, for naught, it was me.

I knew one thing, I wanted to take full advantage of the supernatural healing available, and to believe, as a "thank you" to Jesus for giving his all…for me.

So, I was going to ask for the healing, and receive it without doubting. I raised my arms and relinquished all the analyzing, medical reports, and feeble attempts on my part to try and fight this invisible foe. I would allow God to heal me through Christ.

That was the last day I experienced the ravages of ulcerative colitis. Months later, the results of my routine colonoscopy came back as "totally normal."

I stood in awe of my loving God who really did send His word to heal, and His son who ever lives to make intercession for us. My heart rejoices evermore.

As my strength increased and it was no longer a problem to stay awake while driving home at the end of a shift, Anita, at that time, moved on to another job in town.

I always look back at that situation with fondness for having the chance to make a new friend. To see how God orchestrated such a great way to stay safe while helping someone else in such a way that brought smiles to both of us, is something to be cherished.

Some time after all this happened, I took care of a patient admitted to the hospital with ulcerative colitis and shared my story, to give them the option of reaching up when backed in the corner, as I did. They were so grateful, leaning into Jesus is always a comfort. And by his stripes we most certainly are healed.

CONCLUSION

Hebrews 4:12 NIV

"For the word of God is alive and active. Sharper than any double-edged sword, it penetrates even to the dividing of soul and spirit, joints and marrow; it judges the thoughts and attitudes of the heart."

Ephesians 6:12 Berean Study Bible

"For our struggle is not against flesh and blood, but against the rulers, against the authorities, against the powers of this world's darkness, and against the spiritual forces of evil in the heavenly realms."

Colossians 1:26,27 NIV

"The mystery that had been kept hidden for ages and generations but is now disclosed to the Lord's people. To them God has chosen to make known among the Gentiles, the glorious riches of this mystery, which is Christ in you, the hope of glory."

1 John 1:16 Berean Study Bible

"And we have come to know and come to believe the love that God has for us, God is love, and the one abiding in love abides in God and God abides in Him."

As we equip our minds with the truths and life lessons of God's word, we can walk out on it, fearlessly in His love. Recognizing that our struggles are spiritual in origin and nature, we can now see through the eyes of Jesus, think with the mind of Christ, knowing that the spirit of God, who is in Christ…is in us.

We can be confident that God hears us when we pray.

When the unlovable are loved,

When the unforgiveable are forgiven,

When the unreachable are reached,

When the impossible is believed,

When the unimaginable is received,

When we are filled with joy unspeakable,

That is when we know, Jesus has shown up.

ABOUT THE AUTHOR

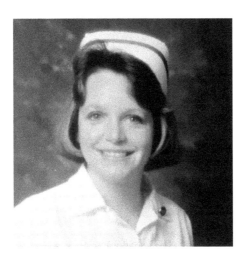

Susan Norris was born in Manchester, NH in 1955 where she was raised with her four siblings. At age 23 she began studying the bible, which began a journey that brought her great joy and freedom. In 1985 she moved to Lexington, KY where she met her husband, Jake Norris, pursued a career in nursing and has retired after 30 years in the field of nursing. After retiring, she was deeply moved to write of those things which she has seen and heard that testify of the living God, so that others may know Him and His son, Jesus. She currently resides in Lebanon, KY where she lives with her husband, and is enjoying the fellowship of their church, their farm, beekeeping, and their little shih tzu, Bella.

.